Sugar Detox for Lazy Girls

Slaying Sugar Cravings with Sass and a Side of Snark

Divine LeRoy

Table of Contents:

Hey there, sugar enthusiasts and fellow lazy girls! I'm Divine LeRoy, your friendly guide to a sugar detox that even the laziest of us can embrace without breaking a sweat (or raiding the chocolate stash). Now, I know what you're thinking – "Divine, a sugar detox? For lazy girls? Isn't that like asking a cat to do the cha-cha?" Well, let me assure you, my dear sweet-toothed comrades, it's not as impossible as it sounds.

In this delightful journey, we're going to navigate the world of sugars with all the grace of a penguin on roller skates. But don't worry, there won't be any stern lectures about the dangers of sugar or intimidating rules that make you want to bury your head in a cupcake graveyard. Nope, we're taking the scenic route, one giggle at a time, as we explore how to tone down our sugar intake without losing our minds (or our taste buds).

So, if you're the type of gal who prefers cozy pajamas over gym clothes and considers a five-minute microwave dinner a gourmet feast, you're in the right place. Together, we're going to learn how to outsmart those sneaky sugars and embrace a simpler, healthier way of life – all while keeping our sense of humor intact.

Buckle up, lazy girls, because we're about to embark on a sugar-detox adventure that's as entertaining as it is empowering. Get ready to kick sugar to the curb without ever breaking a nail (unless, of course, you're trying to open that stubborn pickle jar).

Chapter 1: Sugar, I'm Breaking Up with You

Let's set the stage, shall we? Imagine me, Divine LeRoy, standing in front of my open pantry, glaring at a row of suspiciously tempting snacks. It's a classic showdown – me versus the snacks – and I'm armed with a determination as fierce as a cat defending its cardboard fortress. Oh, the inner turmoil of a lazy girl with an insatiable sweet tooth!

Now, before we dive into this sugar-packed tale, let me assure you that I've had my fair share of sugary escapades. From the late-night rendezvous with a pint of chocolate chip cookie dough ice cream to the passionate embrace of a warm, gooey brownie, I've had a romance with sugar that would put any rom-com to shame. But, as with any great love story, there comes a moment when the protagonist must question whether the relationship is truly a match made in heaven or a recipe for disaster.

Cue the Anecdote: Flashback to a particularly memorable morning where I found myself face-to-face with a bowl of cereal that looked more like a sugar-coated rainbow than breakfast. As I diligently poured milk over the cereal mountains, I couldn't help but marvel at the sheer audacity of calling this concoction "part of a balanced breakfast." Balanced like a unicycle on a tightrope, maybe.

Now, why embark on a sugar detox, you ask? Beyond the obvious reasons – like not wanting my teeth to turn into a dazzling display of sugar art and dodging energy crashes that rival a roller coaster – lies a treasure trove of benefits. Picture it: more stable energy levels than a well-organized spreadsheet, a clearer mind capable of making decisions beyond "cake or cookies," and a newfound appreciation for the natural sweetness that real foods bring to the table.

So, let's raise our imaginary glasses of sparkling water (because we're classy like that) and toast to the grand adventure we're about to undertake. Together, we'll navigate the sugar-infested waters with all the finesse of a swan in tap shoes. And here's the best part: We're going to do it without the fuss, without the complex calculations, and without waving goodbye to our beloved comfort foods.

Drumroll, Please: Lazy girls, it's time to break up with sugar like it's the last piece of awkward dance floor small talk at a party. Picture us tossing sugar packets into the air like confetti as we declare our sugar-free intentions with a flair that rivals a movie star's red carpet entrance.

Now, I know what you're thinking – a sugar detox that's simple, enjoyable, and doesn't involve sacrificing our favorite treats? Sounds about as plausible as finding a unicorn in your backyard. But, dear reader, prepare to be pleasantly surprised. We're about to embark on a sugar detox that's smoother than a perfectly executed hair flip – minus the drama.

So, cozy up in your favorite jammies and get ready to bid adieu to the sugar-coated antics of your past. If breaking up with sugar were an Olympic sport, we'd be taking home the gold, no doubt. So get ready to chuckle your way through this detox journey, because the best way to part ways with sugar is with a side of sass and a dash of humor.

Stay Tuned: Next up, Chapter 2: Sweet Detectives: Unmasking the Hidden Sugars. Because if Sherlock can solve mysteries, we can certainly uncover the sneaky sugars lurking in our everyday foods. Grab your magnifying glass – or, you know, just your reading glasses – and let's solve this sugary whodunit together!

Chapter 2: Sweet Detectives: Unmasking the Hidden Sugars

Welcome, my fellow sugar sleuths, to a chapter that's about to reveal the secrets even the sugariest treats don't want you to know. That's right, we're stepping into our gumshoes and embracing our inner detectives as we dive headfirst into the wild world of hidden sugars. And let me tell you, this is a game more thrilling than a cat chasing a laser pointer.

Picture this: we're undercover agents, armed not with magnifying glasses and trench coats, but with a keen eye for ingredient lists and nutrition labels. Our mission? To expose the sugars that are playing dress-up in foods that parade as innocent. From yogurt cups with more sugar than a dessert buffet to granola bars that are basically candy bars in disguise, we're on the case!

Cue Dramatic Music: Our adventure begins as we step into the grocery store, a battlefield of sugar subterfuge. We'll spot those "healthy" cereals that should come with their own orchestra playing dramatic chords every time they're picked up. And don't even get me started on those cunning condiments that promise a savory experience but secretly sprinkle in sweetness.

Metaphor Time: Think of hidden sugars as the sneaky sidekicks in a spy movie – the ones who pretend to be harmless but are secretly working for the villains. They're the unexpected twist in the plot, the plot twists that keep you guessing till the very end.

But fear not, dear reader, for we're not about to turn this into a Sherlock Holmes marathon. We're the laid-back detectives who prefer solving mysteries while lounging in our favorite recliners. Our mission isn't to intimidate or overwhelm; it's to arm you with knowledge so you can confidently pick out those sugary impostors and send them packing.

Trickster Tactics: And now for the grand finale – our bag of tricks that would make any magician envious. Ever thought of reading the ingredient list backward or squinting at the nutrition label like it's the fine print of a contract? Well, get ready to channel your inner magician because these tricks will help you uncover the hidden sugars with the panache of a seasoned pro.

Think of it this way: unmasking hidden sugars is like playing a game of peek-a-boo with a toddler. Except this time, the toddler is a sugary villain trying to hide behind complicated names like "cane syrup" and "maltodextrin." With our newfound knowledge, we'll see through their disguise and bid them a not-so-fond farewell.

So, sugar detectives, remember this: we're not on a mission to eliminate all sugars from our lives. We're here to be the heroes of our own stories, making informed choices without feeling like we're lost in a maze of sugar-filled mirrors. Get ready to strut through the grocery aisles with a newfound swagger, knowing that you can spot those hidden sugars faster than a squirrel finds a hidden acorn.

Coming Up Next: Chapter 3: Sweet and Emotional: It's Complicated. Because just like unraveling a sugar's true identity, dealing with emotions is an intricate dance that requires its own set of moves. Let's waltz through the world of sugar and feelings, shall we?

Chapter 3: Sweet and Emotional: It's Complicated

Ladies and gentlemen, gather 'round for the greatest soap opera of all time: the one starring our emotions and our favorite leading lady, sugar. It's a tale of intrigue, heartbreak, and unexpected plot twists – and we're here to dive right into the drama with all the finesse of a cat knocking over a vase.

Emotions and sugar consumption, my dear readers, have a relationship that's stickier than a wad of gum on a summer sidewalk. Just when we think we've got it all figured out, they throw us a curveball worthy of the juiciest telenovela. From stress-eating our way through a Netflix binge to celebrating victories with a victory dance straight into a tub of ice cream – our emotions and sugar have perfected the art of synchronized chaos.

Emotion Decoder: Let's be real, we've all been there – the "I had a bad day, I deserve this slice of cake" scenario. But fear not, because we're about to unleash a collection of tactics that are as sharp as a stand-up comedian's wit.

Cravings have a way of striking at the most unexpected times, like a villain revealing their evil plan right before the movie's climax. But don't worry, we're not going to let those cravings lead us astray. We've got tricks up our sleeves, tricks that are so cunning they could outwit even the most devious of cravings.

Comedic Craving Conquerors: Imagine facing a sugar craving with the tenacity of a detective hot on the heels of a suspect. Instead of giving in and tearing into a bag of cookies like a movie villain tearing up a contract, we'll choose to laugh in the face of temptation. Ever tried having a conversation with a craving? It's like talking to that overly dramatic character in a soap opera – and boy, does it make for some entertaining dialogue.

But sugar isn't the only way to manage our emotions, my sugar-detox comrades. Let's get creative! We'll explore stress-relief techniques that don't involve raiding the cookie jar like a bandit. From indulging in a spontaneous dance party to practicing deep-breathing exercises that are as refreshing as a gulp of ice-cold lemonade, we're going to tackle stress with all the flair of a rock star performing to a sold-out crowd.

Stress-Busting Shenanigans: Imagine conquering stress not with a fork and knife, but with laughter and lightheartedness. It's like throwing a surprise party for your stress and watching it transform into a bundle of joy, complete with a party hat and a kazoo.

So, my fellow sugar-craving conquerors, let's navigate the complex waltz between emotions and sugar like the graceful dancers we are. We'll defy the odds, sidestep the drama, and embrace the sweet moments of life without always reaching for the sugar-coated script. Prepare to say "adios" to emotional eating and "hello" to emotional empowerment – all without sacrificing our sense of humor in the process.

Stay Tuned: In Chapter 4, we're diving into the realm of sugar reduction without the drama. Get ready for a showdown with those sneaky sources of sugar that think they can outsmart us. We're about to prove them wrong, one witty tactic at a time!

Chapter 4: Ditching Sugar Without the Drama

Alright, my fellow sugar-detox champions, it's time to roll up our sleeves and tackle sugar reduction with all the gusto of a dog chasing its own tail – minus the chaos, of course. In this chapter, we're going to ditch the sugar without the drama, like a celebrity quietly slipping out of a red carpet event before the paparazzi can catch a glimpse.

Hack Attack: Let's face it, making lifestyle changes can sometimes feel like trying to navigate a labyrinth while blindfolded. But fear not, because we're about to share hacks that are as simple as using a fork instead of chopsticks. We're talking about effortless tricks that'll have you cutting down on sugar like a ninja avoiding booby traps.

Say "goodbye" to overly complicated charts and "hello" to practical strategies that fit perfectly into a lazy girl's daily routine. From swapping sugary sodas for sparkling water that's as refreshing as a dip in a pool on a scorching day to replacing those sugar-laden snacks with alternatives so smart they could graduate summa cum laude from Snack University, we've got you covered.

Alternative Avenue: Now, you might be wondering, "Divine, can I really enjoy life without those saccharine indulgences?" The answer is a resounding "yes," and we're about to prove it to you. We'll introduce you to alternatives that are so delightful, even your taste buds will want to give them a standing ovation.

Picture this: enjoying a bowl of creamy, dreamy banana nice cream that's so easy to whip up, it's practically a magic trick. Or how about a mouthwatering avocado chocolate mousse that's so rich and velvety, you'll forget it's healthy? Yes, my dear reader, the world of guilt-free sweet treats is your oyster, and we're diving in with all the enthusiasm of a kid at a candy store.

Recipe Rendezvous: Oh, and did I mention we're spicing things up with some tongue-in-cheek recipes? Get ready to giggle your way through the creation of treats that taste sinfully decadent but are as virtuous as a well-behaved house cat. You'll be whipping up these goodies faster than you can say "sugar who?"

So, let's kick the sugar drama to the curb and embrace a lifestyle that's as sweet as it is sensible. Get ready to ditch the sugar without feeling like you're missing out on the fun. With our clever hacks and delectable alternatives, you'll be the master of your sugar destiny, sailing smoothly through the land of taste without hitting any sugar-laden icebergs.

Coming Up Next: Chapter 5: Sugar Unleashed: Navigating Social Sweet Spots. Brace yourself for tips and tricks that'll have you confidently sailing through parties, dinners, and gatherings without caving in to sugar's siren call. Get ready to slay those social situations with the charm of a celebrity working the red carpet!

Chapter 5: Sugar Unleashed: Navigating Social Sweet Spots

Hold onto your party hats, because we're about to dive headfirst into the vibrant world of social gatherings, where sugar reigns like a mischievous party crasher. In this chapter, we're stepping into the arena armed with wit, wisdom, and a pinch of sugar-detox magic. Get ready to navigate those social sweet spots like a boss, all while cutting down on sugar and keeping the fun-meter at an all-time high.

Social Symphony: Ah, parties, dinners, and outings – the ultimate proving grounds for anyone aiming to tame their sugar cravings. But fear not, for we're not here to rain on your parade. We're here to help you waltz through these events with all the finesse of a professional dancer, sugar temptations be damned.

Picture this: you, confidently mingling and munching, as if sugar's siren song has been muted by the power of your newfound savvy. From resisting the allure of the dessert table like a seasoned superhero dodging danger to navigating the buffet line with grace and a side of laughter, we've got the playbook to ensure you leave the event triumphant.

Party Diplomacy: Let's be real, the struggle is real when the dessert cart rolls by like a sugar-loaded parade float. But guess what? You've got this. We're tackling the sugar-laden challenges of social gatherings like a dream team that's more formidable than a pack of sugar-hungry squirrels.

But wait, there's more! We're supplying you with savvy tips that'll have you shining brighter than a disco ball on a dance floor. Ever tried mastering the art of small talk with a mocktail in hand, leaving those sugary cocktails in the dust? Get ready to be the life of the party without ever feeling like the sugar police.

Sugary Serenity: Imagine strolling through social events with the grace and confidence of a catwalk model – minus the heels and the paparazzi. Whether it's a swanky dinner or a casual picnic, you're about to glide through them all like a sugar-detox superstar.

So, my dear sugar-savvy readers, get ready to embrace the world of socializing with all the gusto of a karaoke champion. It's time to show those sugar-laden treats who's boss while maintaining the spirit of fun and connection that makes these events memorable. With our arsenal of tips and tricks, you'll breeze through parties and gatherings like a breeze that's just as refreshing as a sugar-free lemonade.

Up Next: Chapter 6: Sweet Moves: Dancing with Health and Fitness. Prepare to explore the powerful synergy between staying active and keeping your inner "lazy girl" well-nurtured. From exercise routines that don't require Olympic training to finding the joy in movement, we're about to make staying active as fun as a sugar-fueled dance party!

Chapter 6: Sweet Moves: Dancing with Health and Fitness

Ladies and gents, it's time to lace up those sneakers and embark on a fitness journey that's as exciting as a roller coaster ride. In this chapter, we're about to dive into the exhilarating world of health and physical activity, all while maintaining the chilled-out spirit of a "lazy girl." So, get ready to put on your best dancing shoes – or, you know, sneakers – as we waltz our way to a healthier, happier you.

Fitness Fusion: Ever heard the saying, "You can't outrun a bad diet"? Well, while that might be true, you can certainly have a blast trying! We're here to explore the wonderful ways that physical activity can help keep those sugar demons at bay. It's like arming yourself with a superhero cape made of endorphins and determination.

Imagine this: you, conquering your day like a warrior on a quest for health, effortlessly shrugging off sugar's seductive whispers. Whether it's a leisurely stroll that rivals a scenic nature walk or a dance party for one in your living room, we're about to make fitness a fun adventure instead of a dreaded chore.

Hilarious Hustle: Now, let's address the elephant in the room: the thought of exercise can be as appealing as brussel sprouts at a pizza party. But fear not, my fellow "lazy girl" enthusiasts, because we've got workouts that are as hilarious as a stand-up comedy show. Say goodbye to the days of strenuous gym sessions that leave you feeling like a deflated balloon – it's time to embrace workouts that make you laugh as much as they make you sweat.

Picture this: attempting a yoga routine that's so relaxed it's practically horizontal, or perhaps a dance workout where the only requirement is moving to the beat (bonus points for groovy dance moves that even your cat would applaud). We're about to prove that fitness can be a joyful experience that keeps those sugar cravings in check, one giggle at a time.

Balanced Bliss: Ah, the fine line between staying active and embracing our inner "lazy girl." It's a delicate dance, like a tightrope walker navigating a world of balance and fun. But guess what? We're here to help you find that equilibrium in a way that's as graceful as a cat stretching after a nap.

Imagine discovering the joy in moving your body without feeling like you're auditioning for the Olympics. Whether it's taking a leisurely bike ride through the park or practicing "chair yoga" (yes, you read that right), we're about to make staying active a part of your life that's as natural as breathing – without the drama.

Coming Up Next: Chapter 7: The Sweet Rewards of a Sugar-Light Future. Get ready to dive into the world of long-term benefits and success stories that will have you embracing a sugar-light lifestyle like a lifelong friend. Stay tuned for a chapter that's as inspiring as it is motivating!

Chapter 7: Sweets for the Future: Glimpse of a Sugar-Light Tomorrow

Prepare to put on your shades, my friends, because we're about to shine a spotlight on the dazzling benefits of embracing a sugar-light lifestyle. In this final chapter, we're diving deep into the crystal-clear waters of a future where sugar no longer holds the reins. Get ready for a glimpse of the sunny days ahead, complete with inspiring tales and a sprinkle of humor that'll leave you smiling like a kid in a candy store.

A Future Less Sweet: Imagine waking up to a world where your energy levels are as steady as a metronome, and your mood is a shining sunbeam that never wanes. That's the promise of reduced sugar intake – a future where you're the captain of your own ship, navigating the seas of life with confidence and vigor.

We're about to explore the long-term benefits that are as golden as a sunrise on a calm ocean. From healthier skin that glows like a summer sunset to a waistline that's as trim as a toplary garden, the rewards of a sugar-light future are waiting for you like hidden treasures on a beach.

Inspiring Sugar Detox Tales: But we're not stopping there, because it's time to introduce you to real-life sugar detox heroes who have triumphed over their sugar-laden pasts. These are the tales of individuals who have shown that saying "no" to sugar doesn't mean saying "no" to joy and satisfaction. Their stories are like guiding stars that light the way to a future free from sugar's grip.

Picture this: the girl next door who swapped her sugar-laden snacks for nutrient-packed powerhouses, or the guy who bid adieu to energy crashes and embraced a life filled with vitality. These are stories of transformation that are as awe-inspiring as a shooting star streaking across the night sky.

Sugar-Light Sunshine: Now, let's talk motivation. Embracing a sugar-light lifestyle isn't about deprivation or restriction; it's about savoring the sweetness of life without being enslaved by the allure of sugar. And yes, we're adding a dash of humor to the mix, because who says healthy living can't be as fun as a stand-up comedy show?

Imagine a future where you're dancing through life like a sunflower in a gentle breeze, your sugar cravings left in the dust like a forgotten memory. It's a future where you're the star of your own show, a show that's equal parts inspiration and entertainment. And guess what? You've got the leading role.

The Grand Finale: As we close this chapter and bid farewell to the journey we've taken together, remember this: a sugar-light future is yours for the taking. It's a future where you're the protagonist, the hero, and the master of your own narrative. So, dear reader, here's to a life that's sweet without being sugary, and a future that's brighter than a fireworks display on a summer night.

Epilogue: A Journey Sweetly Shared: Thank you for joining me on this sugar detox adventure, where we've laughed, learned, and embraced a lifestyle that's as enjoyable as it is nourishing. As you turn the final page of this book, remember that you hold the power to shape your sugar-light future. Now go forth, my sugar-detox superheroes, and savor each moment with all the zest of a zesty lemon!

Conclusion: A Sugar-Light Farewell

And so, dear friends, we come to the final chapter of our sugar detox escapade. It's like bidding adieu to a delightful summer vacation – full of sun-soaked memories, a few mishaps, and a whole lot of laughter. As we close this chapter, let's take a moment to reflect on the journey we've undertaken together and toast to the sweet, sugar-light future that awaits.

Reflecting on the Adventure: From our first steps into the world of sugar reduction to our triumphant battles against sneaky cravings, we've been through it all. We've uncovered hidden sugars like master detectives, swapped sugary treats for scrumptious alternatives, and even waltzed through social events with grace and wit. It's been a journey as rich and diverse as a buffet of flavors, and I hope you've enjoyed every moment as much as I have.

The Heartfelt Lessons: In our quest for a sugar-light future, we've learned that reducing sugar doesn't mean sacrificing joy or satisfaction. It's about making conscious choices that align with our health and happiness – all while keeping our sense of humor intact. We've discovered that we're capable of taming sugar cravings, mastering the art of balance, and finding delight in the simplest of pleasures.

A Sugar-Light Tomorrow: As we bid farewell to the pages of this book, let's step into the future with newfound confidence and excitement. A sugar-light tomorrow is within reach, and it's a world where we're the architects of our own well-being. It's a world where we celebrate victories big and small, knowing that each step taken brings us closer to a life that's vibrant, energetic, and free from sugar's hold.

Stay Sweet, Stay Strong: Remember, dear reader, that a sugar-light lifestyle is a journey, not a destination. There might be moments when temptation knocks on your door, but armed with the knowledge and tools you've gained, you'll be ready to show it the exit. Embrace those moments with grace and a chuckle, and keep moving forward, one step at a time.

With a Grateful Heart: I want to express my heartfelt gratitude for joining me on this adventure. Your commitment to a healthier, happier you is inspiring, and I have no doubt that your sugar-light future will be as bright as the sunniest day. Keep shining, keep smiling, and remember that you've got the power to create a life that's as sweet as can be – with or without the sugar.

Until We Meet Again: As we turn the final page and embark on our individual journeys, let's carry the lessons, laughter, and camaraderie we've shared.

Here's to a future that's sugar-light and filled with joy, vitality, and all the sweetness life has to offer. Until we meet again, my friends, stay sweet, stay strong, and savor every moment. Cheers to a sugar-light farewell and a radiant future ahead!

Appendix: Divine's Delights

Sharing Bonus Recipes and Snack Ideas to Support a Sugar-Light Lifestyle:

Congratulations, savvy reader! You've reached the treasure trove of bonus recipes and snack ideas that'll have you conquering your sugar cravings with style. Get ready to whip up delectable treats that are as nourishing as they are delightful, all while keeping that sugar intake in check. Let's dive into this culinary adventure and create snacks that will leave your taste buds dancing and your energy soaring!

1. Berry Bliss Parfait: Layer Greek yogurt, mixed berries, and a sprinkle of crushed nuts for a parfait that's as vibrant as your sugar-light future. Drizzle with a touch of honey for sweetness that's just right.

2. Guilt-Free Granola Bites: Mix rolled oats, nuts, seeds, and a dash of cinnamon. Form into bite-sized balls and bake until golden. These crunchy delights are perfect for snacking on the go.

3. Sweet Potato Fries with a Twist: Slice sweet potatoes into thin strips, toss with a touch of olive oil, and bake until crispy. Sprinkle with a pinch of sea salt and enjoy a satisfying snack that satisfies both sweet and savory cravings.

4. Cucumber Avocado Sushi Rolls: Lay thin cucumber slices flat, spread avocado on top, and add a hint of lemon juice and a sprinkle of sesame seeds. Roll them up for a refreshing snack that's as elegant as it is nutritious.

5. Chocolate Chia Pudding: Mix chia seeds with almond milk and a touch of unsweetened cocoa powder. Let it sit until it thickens, and voilà – you've got a chocolatey treat that's packed with fiber and goodness.

6. Zesty Roasted Chickpeas: Toss chickpeas with olive oil and your favorite spices (paprika, cumin, and a dash of cayenne work wonders). Roast until crispy, and snack away on these protein-packed delights.

7. Apple Nachos: Slice apples into rounds and arrange them on a plate. Drizzle with a bit of nut butter and sprinkle with chopped nuts, dried fruit, and a touch of cinnamon. It's a snack that's as fun to make as it is to eat.

8. Banana Nice Cream: Blend frozen bananas until creamy and smooth. Top with a handful of crushed nuts and a sprinkle of dark chocolate chips for a dessert that's as dreamy as it is guilt-free.

9. Veggie Dippers with Hummus: Pair carrot sticks, cucumber slices, and bell pepper strips with a generous scoop of homemade hummus. It's a crunchy, satisfying snack that's packed with flavor.

10. DIY Trail Mix: Combine your favorite nuts, seeds, and a sprinkle of unsweetened dried fruit for a personalized trail mix that's tailor-made for your taste buds.

These recipes and snack ideas are your passport to a sugar-light world that's brimming with flavor, vitality, and creativity. So go ahead, embrace your inner chef and whip up these treats with the same enthusiasm you've brought to this sugar detox journey. Here's to a life that's rich in taste, health, and joy – without the sugar drama!

1. "I'm on a sugar-free diet. It's called 'I can't eat that, I'm allergic to feeling terrible.'" - Unknown
2. "Stressed spelled backwards is desserts. Coincidence? I think not!" - Unknown
3. "Life is uncertain. Eat dessert first." - Ernestine Ulmer
4. "Sugar is like a toddler. It's fine in small doses. But if you let it take over, it'll destroy your house." - Unknown
5. "Don't be a slave to sugar; let it be your sweet servant." - Divine LeRoy
6. "Just because you're awake doesn't mean you should stop dreaming of a sugar-light future." - Unknown
7. "Sugar cravings are like your ex – they come back when you're weak." - Unknown
8. "The only drama I enjoy is in my skincare routine, not in my sugar intake." - Unknown
9. "I'm not on a diet; I'm on a 'I enjoy feeling good' journey." - Unknown
10. "Happiness is a balanced diet that includes a little sugar and a lot of laughter." - Unknown
11. "The best things in life are sweet – but they don't always have to come from a sugar packet." - Unknown

12. "Sugar is like a bad ex – it promises happiness but delivers regrets." - Unknown
13. "Don't just count calories; make the calories count with choices that energize and empower you." - Divine LeRoy
14. "Life is too short for cheap chocolate and empty calories." - Unknown
15. "A sugar detox is like a spa day for your body – a little discomfort for a whole lot of rejuvenation." - Unknown
16. "Sweets may be tempting, but the real treat is feeling vibrant and alive." - Divine LeRoy
17. "Health is wealth, and a sugar-light life is the golden ticket." - Unknown
18. "Sugar cravings are like the weather – they pass, and you're left with the clear skies of well-being." - Unknown
19. "Life's sweetness is best savored in moments shared with loved ones, not just in sugary bites." - Unknown
20. "Ditch the sugar, embrace the sparkle. Your body will thank you with every energetic step." - Unknown